OVERCOMING SLEEP PROBLEMS AND INSOMNIA

How to free yourself from sleepless night and stay asleep

Victoria O. Noyes

TABLE OF CONTENT

INTRODUCTION

Sharon was a middle-aged woman who had struggled with insomnia for as long as she could remember. She would lay awake at night, staring at the ceiling, trying to force herself to sleep but never being able to drift off. It was a frustrating and exhausting cycle that left her feeling constantly tired and irritable during the day.

Sharon tried everything she could think of to solve her insomnia. She tried sleeping pills, warm milk before bed, white noise machines, and even relaxation techniques like meditation and deep breathing. None of these seemed to make a difference, and she was starting to feel like she would never be able to get a good night's sleep again.

Finally, Sharon decided to visit a sleep specialist to try to get to the bottom of her insomnia. After discussing her sleep habits and medical history, the specialist suggested that Sharon try cognitive behavioral therapy for insomnia (CBT-I). This is a type of therapy that helps people change their thoughts and behaviors around sleep.

Sharon was skeptical at first, but she was desperate to find a solution, so she decided to give it a try. The therapist worked with her to identify and address any negative thoughts or behaviors that might be contributing to her insomnia. They also helped her develop a consistent sleep routine and taught her relaxation techniques to use before bed.

It was a slow process, but gradually, Sharon started to see improvement in her sleep. She was able to fall asleep more easily and stay asleep throughout the night. She also noticed that she felt more rested and alert during the day.

One of the biggest things that helped Sharon was learning about good sleep hygiene. She realized that she had been making some common mistakes that were disrupting her sleep, such as using her phone or watching TV right before bed, or eating a large meal too close to bedtime.

By making small changes to her routine, she was able to create a more conducive environment for sleep.

Another important factor was addressing her stress and anxiety. Sharon had a lot on her plate, and she realized that she was bringing those worries to bed with her. The therapy helped her learn how to manage her stress and worry in a healthy way, so she was able to relax and let go of those thoughts before bed.

It wasn't an overnight fix, but with time and practice, Sharon was able to overcome her insomnia and get the restful sleep she had been longing for. She was grateful to the therapist for helping her identify and address the root causes of her sleep problems, and she felt like a new person with the energy and clarity that a good night's sleep provided.

If you're struggling with insomnia like Sharon was, it's important to know that you're not alone and that there are effective treatments available.

Don't be afraid to seek help and try different strategies until you find what works for you. It may take some time and effort, but the rewards of a good night's sleep are well worth it.

You can also overcome insomnia just the way Sharon did. Journey with me to discover the truth that was discussed with her by the therapist which eventually helped her.

CHAPTER 1

WHAT INSOMNIA IS AND ITS CAUSES

Insomnia is a common sleep disorder that involves difficulty falling asleep, staying asleep, or getting restful sleep. It can have a variety of causes, including stress, anxiety, medical conditions, and certain medications.

The concept of insomnia dates back to ancient times. In ancient Greek and Roman literature, there are references to people having difficulty falling asleep and to the use of sedatives to treat insomnia. In traditional Chinese medicine, insomnia is believed to be caused by an imbalance of yin and yang in the body.

Insomnia was first formally recognized as a medical condition in the late 19th century. In the 20th century, research on the causes and treatment of insomnia increased, leading to the development of various therapies and medications for the disorder. Today, insomnia is a common condition that affects millions of people around the world. It is often treated with a combination of lifestyle changes, therapy, and medication.

There are many potential causes of insomnia, including:

- Stress: Stressful events or situations can make it difficult to fall asleep or stay asleep.

- Anxiety: Anxiety disorders can cause racing thoughts and make it difficult to relax and fall asleep.

- Depression: Depression can cause feelings of hopelessness and lack of energy, which can make it difficult to fall asleep or stay asleep.

- Medical conditions: Certain medical conditions, such as chronic pain, asthma, or acid reflux, can cause insomnia.

- Medications: Some medications, such as antidepressants, stimulants, and decongestants, can disrupt sleep.

- Poor sleep hygiene: Habits such as watching TV or using electronic devices before bed, consuming caffeine or alcohol before sleep, or having an irregular sleep schedule can all contribute to insomnia.

- Age: Insomnia becomes more common as people get older, and older adults are more likely to experience difficulty falling asleep and staying asleep.

- Shift work: Working non-traditional hours or frequently changing work schedules can disrupt the body's natural sleep-wake cycle and lead to insomnia.

- Women's health: Hormonal changes, such as those that occur during pregnancy, menopause, and menstrual cycles, can contribute to insomnia.

- Environmental factors: Noise, light, and temperature can all affect sleep quality and contribute to insomnia.

- Genetics: Insomnia can run in families, suggesting that there may be a genetic component to the disorder.

How stress can cause insomnia:
Stress is a common cause of insomnia and can have a significant impact on sleep quality. Stress activates the body's "fight or flight" response, which releases stress hormones such as cortisol and adrenaline. These hormones can disrupt the body's natural sleep-wake cycle, making it difficult to fall asleep or stay asleep.

Stress can also cause racing thoughts and make it difficult to relax and fall asleep. When we are under stress, our minds may be preoccupied with worries and concerns, which can keep us awake at night. Additionally, stress can cause physical symptoms such as muscle tension and pain, which can make it difficult to get comfortable and sleep soundly.

Stress can also disrupt sleep patterns by causing us to lie awake at night worrying about things that need to be done or events that may happen in the future. This can make it difficult to fall asleep or stay asleep, as our minds are active and we are unable to relax.

Furthermore, stress can lead to irregular sleep schedules. For example, if we are under a lot of stress, we may find ourselves staying up late to finish tasks or meet deadlines, which can lead to insomnia. Similarly, if we are stressed, we may have difficulty waking up in the morning, which can affect our sleep-wake cycle and lead to insomnia.

There are also indirect ways in which stress can contribute to insomnia. For example, if we are under a lot of stress, we may be more likely to engage in unhealthy habits such as consuming caffeine or alcohol before bed, which can disrupt sleep. Similarly, we may be less likely to prioritize self-care and engage in relaxation techniques such as meditation or yoga, which can help us sleep better.

In summary, stress is a common cause of insomnia and can have a significant impact on sleep quality. Stress activates the body's "fight or flight" response, which releases stress hormones that can disrupt the body's natural sleep-wake cycle. Stress can also cause racing thoughts and physical symptoms such as muscle tension and pain, which can make it difficult to sleep soundly. Additionally, stress can lead to irregular sleep schedules and disrupt sleep patterns by causing us to lie awake at night worrying. Finally, stress can also contribute to insomnia indirectly by leading to unhealthy habits and a lack of self-care.

How anxiety can cause insomnia:
Anxiety and insomnia often go hand in hand, with one condition often exacerbating the other.

Anxiety can lead to insomnia in a number of ways, and it is important to understand these mechanisms in order to effectively treat both conditions.

One of the most common ways that anxiety can lead to insomnia is through racing thoughts and worry. When a person is anxious, their mind may become fixated on certain thoughts or concerns, making it difficult to calm down and relax enough to fall asleep. These racing thoughts can keep a person awake at night, making it difficult to get the rest they need.

Another way that anxiety can contribute to insomnia is through physical symptoms. Anxiety can cause a range of physical symptoms, including increased heart rate, difficulty breathing, and muscle tension. These symptoms can make it difficult to relax and fall asleep, especially if they are severe.

In addition to these direct effects on sleep, anxiety can also lead to insomnia through behaviors and habits that disrupt sleep. For example, people who are anxious may engage in activities such as checking their phone or watching TV late at night, which can disrupt the body's natural sleep-wake cycle. They may also be more prone to caffeine or alcohol consumption, which can interfere with sleep.

Treatment for anxiety-induced insomnia typically involves addressing the underlying anxiety as well as addressing any sleep-specific behaviors and habits that may be contributing to the problem. Therapy, such as cognitive-behavioral therapy (CBT) or relaxation techniques, can be helpful in managing anxiety and improving sleep. Additionally, establishing a consistent sleep routine and avoiding stimulating activities before bedtime can be beneficial. In some cases, medication may also be prescribed to help manage anxiety or improve sleep.

It is important to seek treatment for both anxiety and insomnia, as they can have a negative impact on overall health and well-being. Left untreated, anxiety and insomnia can lead to a range of problems, including difficulty functioning during the day, impaired memory and concentration, and an increased risk of physical health problems such as high blood pressure and cardiovascular disease.

How depression can cause insomnia:
Depression and insomnia are often closely related, with one condition often leading to the other. Depression can cause insomnia, and insomnia can also exacerbate or prolong depression. It is important to address both conditions in order to achieve optimal mental health.

Depression is a common and serious mental health disorder that is characterized by persistent feelings of sadness, hopelessness, and a lack of interest or pleasure in activities. It can also manifest as physical symptoms such as changes in appetite and sleep patterns, fatigue, and difficulty concentrating. Depression can be caused by a variety of factors, including genetics, stress, life events, and underlying medical conditions.

Insomnia is a common sleep disorder that is characterized by difficulty falling asleep or staying asleep, or waking up too early in the morning. It can also lead to non-restorative sleep, where an individual may feel tired or unrefreshed even after sleeping for a sufficient amount of time. Insomnia can be caused by a variety of factors, including medical conditions, medications, and lifestyle factors such as caffeine and alcohol consumption, irregular sleep schedule, and stress.

Depression and insomnia often occur together and can have a reciprocal relationship. Depression can lead to insomnia, as the negative thoughts and feelings associated with depression can make it difficult to fall asleep or stay asleep. Depression can also cause changes in sleep patterns, such as oversleeping or difficulty waking up in the morning. In addition, certain medications used to treat depression can have sleep-related side effects.

Insomnia can also exacerbate or prolong depression, as poor sleep quality can lead to increased fatigue, difficulty concentrating, and irritability. These symptoms can make it difficult to carry out daily activities and can further contribute to feelings of hopelessness and helplessness. In addition, the stress and frustration of trying to get a good night's sleep can also contribute to a negative mood.

There are several treatment options available for individuals experiencing both depression and insomnia. It is important to seek help from a mental health professional, such as a therapist or a psychiatrist, for treatment of depression. Treatment options for depression may include medication, therapy, or a combination of both.

Medications used to treat depression include selective serotonin reuptake inhibitors (SSRIs), serotonin-norepinephrine reuptake inhibitors

(SNRIs), and tricyclic antidepressants. These medications work by increasing the levels of certain chemicals in the brain, such as serotonin and norepinephrine, which are involved in mood regulation. It is important to work closely with a healthcare provider to determine the best medication and dosage for an individual's needs.

Therapy, such as cognitive behavioral therapy (CBT), can be an effective treatment for both depression and insomnia. CBT focuses on identifying and changing negative thought patterns and behaviors that contribute to the development and maintenance of depression and insomnia. It can help individuals develop healthy sleep habits and coping strategies for managing negative thoughts and emotions.

In addition to medication and therapy, there are also lifestyle changes that can help improve both depression and insomnia. These may include maintaining a regular sleep schedule, creating a relaxing bedtime routine, reducing caffeine and alcohol consumption, and engaging in regular physical activity. It may also be helpful to limit screen time before bed and create a comfortable sleep environment, such as keeping the bedroom cool and dark.

In summary, depression and insomnia are closely related, with one condition often leading to the other. It is important to address both conditions in order to achieve optimal mental health. Treatment options for depression and insomnia may include medication, therapy, and lifestyle changes.

How medical condition can cause insomnia: Insomnia is a common sleep disorder that can be caused by a variety of factors, including medical conditions such as chronic pain, asthma, and acid reflux. Let's take a closer look at how each of these conditions can contribute to insomnia.

Chronic pain is a persistent type of pain that lasts for weeks, months, or even years. It can be caused by a variety of conditions, including arthritis, fibromyalgia, and back injuries.

Chronic pain can be physically and emotionally draining, and it can make it difficult to fall asleep or stay asleep. This is because pain activates the body's stress response, releasing stress hormones such as adrenaline and cortisol. These hormones can make it difficult to relax and fall asleep, leading to insomnia.

Asthma is a respiratory disorder characterized by inflammation and narrowing of the airways, which can make it difficult to breathe. Asthma attacks can be triggered by a variety of factors, including allergens, exercise, and cold air. During an asthma attack, the airways become constricted and produce excess mucus, which can make it difficult to breathe and sleep. Asthma attacks can also cause coughing, wheezing, and shortness of breath, which can further disrupt sleep.

Acid reflux, also known as gastroesophageal reflux disease (GERD), is a condition in which stomach acid flows back into the esophagus, causing heartburn and other symptoms. Acid reflux can be caused by a variety of factors, including diet, lifestyle, and certain medications. Acid reflux can be especially problematic at night, as lying down can allow stomach acid to flow back into the esophagus more easily. This can lead to symptoms such as heartburn, chest pain, and difficulty swallowing, which can make it difficult to fall asleep or stay asleep.

In addition to these medical conditions, other factors such as stress, anxiety, and depression can also contribute to insomnia. These conditions can activate the body's stress response, making it difficult to relax and fall asleep. They can also cause racing thoughts and worry, which can further disrupt sleep.

Treatment for insomnia caused by medical conditions such as chronic pain, asthma, and acid reflux often involves addressing the underlying condition. This can involve medications to control pain, asthma, or acid reflux, as well as lifestyle changes such as diet and exercise. In some cases, behavioral therapies such as cognitive behavioral therapy (CBT) can also be helpful in addressing insomnia. CBT is a type of therapy that focuses on changing negative thought patterns and behaviors that contribute to insomnia, and it can be effective in improving sleep.

It's important to note that insomnia can have a serious impact on overall health and well-being. Chronic insomnia can lead to fatigue, difficulty concentrating, and an increased risk of accidents and injuries. It can also contribute to other health problems such as heart disease, diabetes, and obesity.

How medication can cause insomnia:
Insomnia is a common sleep disorder characterized by difficulty falling asleep, staying asleep, or getting restful sleep. It can be caused by a variety of factors, including medical conditions, lifestyle habits, and medications. Some medications, such as antidepressants, stimulants, and decongestants, can cause insomnia as a side effect.

Antidepressants are medications used to treat depression and other mental health conditions. They work by adjusting the levels of certain chemicals in the brain called neurotransmitters, which play a role in mood and behavior. Some common types of antidepressants include selective serotonin reuptake inhibitors (SSRIs), serotonin-norepinephrine reuptake inhibitors (SNRIs), and tricyclic antidepressants (TCAs). While these medications can be effective in treating depression, they can also cause insomnia as a side effect.

SSRIs, such as fluoxetine (Prozac), paroxetine (Paxil), and sertraline (Zoloft), can cause insomnia by increasing the levels of serotonin in the brain. Serotonin is a neurotransmitter that helps regulate sleep-wake cycles, and increased levels can make it harder to fall asleep or stay asleep. SNRIs, such as venlafaxine (Effexor) and duloxetine (Cymbalta), can also cause insomnia by affecting the levels of both serotonin and norepinephrine in the brain. Norepinephrine is another neurotransmitter that helps regulate sleep-wake cycles, and increased levels can interfere with sleep.

TCAs, such as amitriptyline (Elavil) and nortriptyline (Pamelor), can also cause insomnia as a side effect. TCAs work by inhibiting the reuptake of certain neurotransmitters, including norepinephrine and serotonin, which can lead to increased levels of these neurotransmitters in the brain and interfere with sleep.

Stimulants are medications that increase activity in the central nervous system and are often used to treat conditions such as attention deficit hyperactivity disorder (ADHD) and narcolepsy. Some common stimulants include amphetamines, such as Adderall and Ritalin, and methylphenidate, such as Concerta and ritalin. While these medications can be effective in treating these conditions, they can also cause insomnia as a side effect.

Stimulants work by increasing the levels of certain neurotransmitters, including dopamine and norepinephrine, in the brain. These neurotransmitters are involved in the regulation of sleep-wake cycles, and increased levels can make it harder to fall asleep or stay asleep. Additionally, stimulants can cause feelings of alertness and increased energy, which can make it difficult to relax and fall asleep.

Decongestants are medications used to relieve nasal congestion and other symptoms of allergies and the common cold. They work by narrowing the blood vessels in the nasal passages and reducing swelling, which helps to reduce congestion. Some common decongestants include pseudoephedrine, found in medications such as Sudafed, and phenylephrine, found in medications such as Sudafed PE. While these medications can be effective in relieving nasal congestion, they can also cause insomnia as a side effect.

Decongestants work by stimulating the central nervous system, which can lead to increased alertness and difficulty falling asleep. They can also cause side effects such as jitters, nervousness, and increased heart rate, which can make it difficult to relax and fall asleep.

If you are taking a medication that is causing insomnia, it is important to talk to your healthcare provider about your sleep difficulties.

How poor sleep hygiene can cause insomnia:
Poor sleep hygiene refers to habits and behaviors that disrupt or interfere with a person's ability to fall asleep and stay asleep throughout the night. These habits can lead to insomnia, a sleep disorder characterized by difficulty falling asleep, staying asleep, or both. Insomnia can have serious consequences, including difficulty functioning during the day, decreased productivity, and an increased risk of developing other health problems.

One of the main factors that can contribute to poor sleep hygiene is a lack of consistent sleep schedule. Going to bed and waking up at the same time every day helps to regulate the body's natural sleep-wake cycle, also known as the circadian rhythm. When this rhythm is disrupted, it can be more difficult to fall asleep and stay asleep.

Another factor that can impact sleep hygiene is the environment in which a person sleeps. The bedroom should be a peaceful, comfortable space that is conducive to sleep. Noise, light, and temperature can all affect sleep quality. It is important to eliminate as much noise and light as possible, and to maintain a comfortable temperature in the bedroom.

The use of electronic devices, such as phones, tablets, and computers, can also interfere with sleep hygiene. The blue light emitted by these devices can suppress the production of melatonin, a hormone that helps regulate sleep. It is recommended to avoid screens for at least an hour before bedtime, or to use blue light blocking filters to minimize the impact on sleep.

Caffeine, alcohol, and tobacco use can also affect sleep quality. Caffeine is a stimulant that can interfere with the body's ability to relax and fall asleep. Alcohol may help a person fall asleep initially, but it can disrupt sleep later in the night. Tobacco use can also interfere with sleep, as nicotine is a stimulant that can cause sleep disturbances.

Stress and anxiety can also play a role in poor sleep hygiene and insomnia. It is important to manage stress and find ways to relax before bedtime, such as through relaxation techniques like meditation or deep breathing.

It is also important to maintain a healthy diet and exercise routine, as these can contribute to overall sleep quality. Avoiding heavy, fatty meals late at night and engaging in regular physical activity can help improve sleep.

In summary, poor sleep hygiene can lead to insomnia by disrupting the body's natural sleep-wake cycle, affecting the sleep environment, interfering with the use of electronic devices, and impacting the consumption of caffeine, alcohol, and tobacco. Stress and poor diet and exercise habits can also play a role. By addressing these factors and adopting healthy sleep habits, it is possible to improve sleep hygiene and overcome insomnia.

How age can cause insomnia:
Insomnia is a common sleep disorder that can affect people of all ages. However, age alone can be a significant factor in the development of insomnia. As we get older, our bodies and minds go through various changes that can disrupt our sleep patterns and make it more difficult to fall asleep or stay asleep throughout the night.

One of the main reasons that age can cause insomnia is due to changes in our sleep patterns and sleep needs as we age. As we get older, our bodies produce less melatonin, a hormone that helps regulate sleep. This can make it harder to fall asleep and stay asleep. Additionally, older adults often have more medical conditions that can disrupt sleep, such as chronic pain, sleep apnea, and restless leg syndrome.

Another factor that can contribute to insomnia as we age is lifestyle changes. As we get older, we may experience changes in our work schedule or daily routine that can disrupt our sleep patterns. For example, if we retire or change jobs, we may find ourselves going to bed at different times or waking up at different times than we are used to. Additionally, older adults may have more responsibilities and stressors that can keep them awake at night, such as caring for a sick family member or worrying about financial issues.

There are also several physiological changes that can occur as we age that can affect our sleep. For example, older adults may have a harder time falling asleep because they have a harder time regulating their body temperature. This can be due to a decrease in the production of hormones such as estrogen and testosterone, which help regulate body temperature. Additionally, older adults may have a harder time staying asleep because they are more likely to experience sleep-disrupting medical conditions such as sleep apnea, which is a condition in which a person stops breathing briefly during sleep.

Another factor that can contribute to insomnia in older adults is the use of medications. Many older adults take multiple medications for various medical conditions, and some of these medications can have side effects that disrupt sleep. For example, some medications used to treat high blood pressure or anxiety can cause insomnia, while others can cause excessive drowsiness or sleepiness. It is important for older adults to talk to their healthcare provider about any sleep problems they are experiencing and to discuss the potential impact of their medications on their sleep.

In conclusion, age can cause insomnia due to changes in sleep patterns and needs, lifestyle changes, physiological changes, and the use of medications. Treatment may include lifestyle changes, such as establishing a consistent sleep schedule and creating a relaxing bedtime routine, and may also include medications or setting a good night's sleep.

How shift work can cause insomnia:
Shift work refers to a work schedule that involves rotating or irregular work hours, typically outside the traditional 9-to-5 workday. This can include evening, night, or early morning shifts. While shift work can offer flexibility and the opportunity to earn additional income, it can also have negative impacts on an individual's sleep patterns and overall health. One common issue that shift workers may face is insomnia, a disorder characterized by difficulty falling asleep or staying asleep. In this article, we will explore how shift work alone can cause insomnia and some strategies for managing this condition.

One reason shift work may lead to insomnia is that it disrupts the body's natural circadian rhythm, the internal biological clock that regulates sleep-wake cycles. The body is programmed to be awake during the day and asleep at night, and this rhythm is regulated by various hormones and neurotransmitters. When an individual works at night or on rotating shifts, they may be required to sleep during the day when their body is programmed to be awake, leading to difficulty falling asleep or staying asleep.

In addition to disrupting the body's natural circadian rhythm, shift work may also contribute to insomnia by increasing stress and anxiety. Shift work often requires working during non-traditional hours, which can lead to social isolation and a lack of support from family and friends. Shift workers may also feel pressure to perform well on the job, leading to increased stress and anxiety. These factors can make it difficult to relax and fall asleep, leading to insomnia.

There are several strategies that shift workers can use to manage insomnia and improve their sleep quality. One strategy is to maintain a consistent sleep schedule as much as possible. This means going to bed and waking up at the same time every day, even on days off. Establishing a relaxing bedtime routine, such as taking a warm bath or reading a book, can also help prepare the body for sleep.

Another strategy is to create a sleep-friendly environment by reducing distractions and noise in the bedroom and keeping the room at a comfortable temperature. Using a white noise machine or earplugs may also help to block out external noise and promote sleep.

In addition to these strategies, shift workers may also benefit from using relaxation techniques, such as deep breathing or progressive muscle relaxation, to help calm the mind and body before sleep. Exercise, especially during the day, can also improve sleep quality by promoting relaxation and helping to regulate the body's natural sleep-wake cycle.

It is also important for shift workers to pay attention to their diet and hydration. Avoiding caffeine, alcohol, and large meals close to bedtime can help improve sleep quality. Staying hydrated by drinking plenty of water throughout the day can also help promote sleep.

In conclusion, shift work alone can cause insomnia due to its disruption of the body's natural circadian rhythm and increased stress and anxiety. However, by following some simple strategies, such as maintaining a consistent sleep schedule, creating a sleep-friendly environment, using relaxation techniques, and paying attention to diet and hydration, shift workers can improve their sleep quality and manage insomnia.

How women's health can cause insomnia:
Insomnia is a common sleep disorder that can significantly impact a person's quality of life. It is characterized by difficulty falling asleep,

staying asleep, or getting restful sleep. Insomnia can be caused by a variety of factors, including psychological and physiological issues, as well as environmental and lifestyle factors.

One area that is often overlooked when it comes to insomnia is women's health. There are several ways in which women's health can cause or contribute to insomnia, and understanding these factors can help women seeking treatment for their sleep problems.

One common cause of insomnia in women is hormonal fluctuations. The menstrual cycle, pregnancy, and menopause are all times when a woman's hormones are in flux, and these changes can affect sleep patterns. For example, during the luteal phase of the menstrual cycle (the time between ovulation and the start of the next period), levels of the hormone progesterone rise. This can lead to an increase in body temperature and a decrease in the production of melatonin, a hormone that helps regulate sleep.

As a result, women may experience difficulty falling or staying asleep during this time.

Pregnancy can also cause insomnia, particularly in the first and third trimesters. During pregnancy, levels of the hormone progesterone increase, which can lead to sleep problems. In addition, the growing uterus can put pressure on the bladder and cause frequent urination, which can disrupt sleep. Finally, pregnancy can also cause physical discomfort, such as back pain or heartburn, which can make it difficult to sleep.

Menopause is another time when hormonal changes can cause insomnia. As a woman approaches menopause, her levels of estrogen and progesterone begin to decline, which can lead to sleep problems. In addition, hot flashes and night sweats, which are common during menopause, can also disrupt sleep.

Other women's health issues that can cause insomnia include premenstrual syndrome (PMS), endometriosis, and uterine fibroids. PMS is a group of physical and emotional symptoms that occur in the week or two before a woman's period. These symptoms can include mood changes, bloating, and fatigue, all of which can interfere with sleep. Endometriosis is a condition in which the tissue that lines the uterus grows outside of the uterus, and it can cause chronic pain and discomfort that can disrupt sleep. Uterine fibroids are non-cancerous tumors that grow in the uterus, and they can cause discomfort and pressure that can make it difficult to sleep.

There are also several medical conditions that can affect women's sleep, including sleep apnea, restless leg syndrome, and chronic pain. Sleep apnea is a disorder in which a person's breathing is briefly interrupted during sleep, and it can cause snoring and wakefulness. Restless leg syndrome is a disorder in which a person experiences an irresistible urge to move their legs, often due to discomfort or tingling sensations. Chronic pain, such as that caused by arthritis or fibromyalgia, can also disrupt sleep.

In conclusion, women's health can be a significant factor in the development of insomnia. Hormonal fluctuations, medical conditions, and other health issues can all contribute to sleep problems in women. Understanding the specific causes of insomnia can help women seeking treatment for their sleep problems.

How environmental factors can cause insomnia:
Insomnia is a common sleep disorder characterized by difficulty falling or staying asleep, or by experiencing non-restorative sleep. It can be caused by a variety of factors, including environmental factors such as noise, light, temperature, and other disruptions to the sleep environment.

Noise can be a major contributor to insomnia. It can come from a variety of sources, including traffic, neighbors, pets, or even sounds within the home such as a ticking clock or creaky floorboards. Loud or sudden noises can disrupt sleep, causing a person to wake up or have difficulty falling back asleep. Even low-level noise can interfere with sleep, especially if it is unexpected or irregular. It is important to create a quiet and peaceful sleep environment in order to minimize the impact of noise on sleep.

Light can also affect sleep quality. Exposure to bright light during the day can help regulate the body's sleep-wake cycle, but exposure to light at night can disrupt sleep. The blue light emitted by electronic devices such as smartphones, laptops, and TVs can interfere with the production of melatonin, a hormone that helps regulate sleep. It is important to avoid screens and other sources of blue light for at least an hour before bed, and to create a dark sleep environment by using blackout curtains or an eye mask.

Temperature is another important factor in sleep quality. The body's internal temperature naturally drops during sleep, which helps to initiate and maintain sleep. A sleep environment that is too hot or too cold can disrupt this process, leading to difficulty falling or staying asleep. It is generally recommended to keep the bedroom cool, with a temperature of around 65°F (18°C) being ideal for sleep.

Other disruptions to the sleep environment can also cause insomnia. These can include uncomfortable bedding or a mattress that is too hard or too soft, an unruly sleep partner, or a cluttered or cluttered bedroom. It is important to create a comfortable and relaxing sleep environment in order to promote good sleep quality.

In conclusion, environmental factors alone can cause insomnia. Noise, light, temperature, and other disruptions to the sleep environment can all affect sleep quality and lead to difficulty falling or staying asleep. By creating a quiet, dark, and comfortable sleep environment, it is possible to improve sleep quality and reduce the risk of insomnia.

How genetics can cause insomnia

Insomnia is a common sleep disorder characterized by difficulty falling or staying asleep, or waking up too early and being unable to fall back asleep. It can have a significant impact on an individual's quality of life and can lead to a range of physical and mental health problems. While there are many potential causes of insomnia, including environmental, psychological, and medical factors, genetics can also play a role in its development.

There is evidence that certain genetic variations may increase the risk of developing insomnia. For example, research has identified genetic variations in the genes that regulate the body's internal clock, known as the circadian rhythm, that are associated with a higher risk of insomnia. The circadian rhythm is a natural process that helps regulate sleep-wake cycles, and disruptions to this process can lead to problems with sleep.

Other genetic variations that have been linked to insomnia include those in the genes that regulate the production and metabolism of neurotransmitters, such as serotonin and dopamine, which are involved in sleep regulation. Some studies have also found that people with certain genetic variations in the genes involved in the stress response system may be more likely to develop insomnia.

It is worth noting that while genetics can contribute to the development of insomnia, they are not the only factor. Environmental and lifestyle factors, such as work schedule, diet, and stress levels, can also play a role. Additionally, certain medical conditions, such as anxiety and depression, can cause insomnia.

It is also important to note that genetics is a complex field and that the relationship between genetics and insomnia is still not fully understood. More research is needed to fully understand the role that genetics plays in the development of insomnia and to identify specific genetic variations that may increase the risk.

Despite the limited understanding of the role of genetics in insomnia, there are steps that individuals can take to improve their sleep. These include establishing a consistent sleep routine, creating a sleep-friendly environment, and adopting healthy sleep habits such as avoiding caffeine and alcohol before bed, and getting regular exercise. In some cases, individuals with insomnia may also benefit from seeking treatment from a healthcare professional, such as a sleep specialist or a mental health professional.

In summary, genetics can play a role in the development of insomnia, although the exact relationship between genetics and insomnia is still not fully understood. While genetics can contribute to the risk of developing insomnia, environmental and lifestyle factors, as well as medical conditions, can also be involved. To improve sleep, individuals can adopt healthy sleep habits and seek treatment if needed.

CHAPTER 2

SYMPTOMS OF INSOMNIA

Insomnia is a sleep disorder that is characterized by difficulty falling asleep, staying asleep, or getting restful sleep. People with insomnia may have one or more of the following symptoms:

Difficulty falling asleep: This is the most common symptom of insomnia and refers to the inability to fall asleep within a reasonable amount of time. People with insomnia may lie awake for long periods of time trying to fall asleep, or they may fall asleep but wake up frequently throughout the night.

There are several reasons why people with insomnia might have difficulty falling asleep alone. One reason is that they may have racing thoughts or worry, which can make it difficult to relax and fall asleep. Another reason is that they may have physical discomfort or pain, which can make it difficult to get comfortable in bed and fall asleep. Additionally, people with insomnia may have a disrupted sleep-wake cycle, which can make it difficult to fall asleep at the same time every night.

There are several strategies that can help people with insomnia fall asleep more easily. One strategy is to establish a consistent sleep routine, which can help regulate the body's natural sleep-wake cycle. This might involve going to bed at the same time every night, setting a consistent wake-up time, and avoiding napping during the day. Other strategies include creating a relaxing bedtime routine, such as reading or listening to soothing music, and reducing or eliminating caffeine and alcohol consumption, especially close to bedtime.

Another effective strategy for people with insomnia is to practice relaxation techniques, such as deep breathing, progressive muscle relaxation, or mindfulness meditation. These techniques can help calm the mind and body, making it easier to fall asleep.

It is also important for people with insomnia to address any underlying causes of their difficulty falling asleep, such as physical discomfort, stress, or anxiety. Working with a healthcare provider or sleep specialist can help identify and address these underlying causes, and may involve the use of medication or other treatment options.

Overall, difficulty falling asleep alone is a common symptom of insomnia, and there are various strategies and treatments that can help people with insomnia get a good night's sleep. By establishing a consistent sleep routine, practicing relaxation techniques, and addressing any underlying causes, people with insomnia can improve their sleep and reduce their difficulty falling asleep alone.

Waking up frequently during the night:
People with insomnia may wake up several
times during the night and have difficulty falling
back asleep. This can lead to a feeling of being
rested in the morning.

Insomnia is a common sleep disorder that can
cause difficulty falling asleep, staying asleep, or
both. One of the primary symptoms of insomnia
is waking up frequently during the night. People
with insomnia may wake up several times during
the night or may wake up for long periods of
time and have difficulty falling back asleep.

There are many potential causes of insomnia,
including stress, anxiety, depression, medication
side effects, and poor sleep hygiene. People with
insomnia may also have underlying health
conditions, such as sleep apnea or restless leg
syndrome, that contribute to their sleep
problems.

Waking up frequently during the night can have
significant negative impacts on daily life,

including fatigue, difficulty concentrating, and reduced productivity. It can also lead to irritability and difficulty functioning in social situations.

Waking up too early: People with insomnia may wake up earlier than they want to and be unable to fall back asleep. This can lead to feelings of fatigue and sleepiness during the day.

Waking up too early alone is a common symptom of insomnia, a sleep disorder that affects millions of people around the world. Insomnia is characterized by difficulty falling asleep or staying asleep, resulting in poor sleep quality and daytime fatigue. People with insomnia may wake up frequently during the night or wake up too early and be unable to fall back asleep.

One of the main causes of insomnia is stress and anxiety. When we are under stress or worrying about something, our bodies become tense and our minds become racing, making it difficult to relax and fall asleep. This can lead to early morning awakenings, as our bodies are still in a state of alertness and not fully rested.

Waking up too early alone can be frustrating and disruptive to our daily routines, as it can leave us feeling tired and unable to function properly throughout the day. It can also lead to a cycle of poor sleep, as we may lay awake in bed worrying about not being able to fall back asleep, further exacerbating the problem.

It is important to remember that insomnia is a treatable condition and that seeking help can lead to improved sleep and overall health.

Difficulty staying asleep: People with insomnia may fall asleep easily but wake up frequently during the night and have difficulty falling back asleep. This can lead to feelings of fatigue and sleepiness during the day.

People with sleep maintenance insomnia may have trouble falling asleep initially, but once they do fall asleep, they may wake up frequently throughout the night and have difficulty returning to sleep. This can lead to a cycle of poor sleep quality, as the individual may feel tired and restless during the day due to insufficient sleep.

Treatment for sleep maintenance insomnia typically involves a combination of lifestyle changes and medication. Lifestyle changes may include establishing a regular sleep schedule, practicing relaxation techniques such as meditation or deep breathing, and avoiding caffeine and alcohol close to bedtime. Medications, such as sedatives or melatonin, may also be prescribed to help with sleep.

Poor sleep quality: People with insomnia may sleep for a sufficient amount of time, but the sleep is often light and not restful. They may wake up feeling tired and unrefreshed.

Poor sleep quality can have serious consequences for an individual's physical and mental health. It can lead to increased risk of chronic conditions such as heart disease, diabetes, and obesity, and can also contribute to mental health problems such as anxiety and depression. Treatment options may include lifestyle changes, such as establishing a consistent bedtime routine and avoiding screens before bed.

Daytime fatigue: People with insomnia may experience fatigue and sleepiness during the day, even after a full night's sleep. This can affect their ability to concentrate and perform daily tasks.

Difficulty concentrating: Insomnia can affect a person's ability to concentrate and perform tasks, leading to problems at work or school.

Mood changes: Insomnia can cause irritability, mood swings, and difficulty managing stress.

Mood changes associated with insomnia can include feelings of sadness, irritability, frustration, and anxiety. These changes in mood can be caused by a lack of restful sleep, which can lead to a decline in overall physical and mental health. Insomnia can also lead to a decrease in productivity and an increase in the risk of accidents or injuries, as well as a greater risk of developing other mental health conditions, such as depression or anxiety.

There are several factors that can contribute to mood changes in people with insomnia. One of the most common is a disrupted sleep-wake cycle, which can be caused by a variety of factors, such as work schedule changes, jet lag, or sleep disorders such as sleep apnea. Stress and anxiety can also play a role in insomnia and mood changes, as can physical and mental health conditions, such as chronic pain, depression, or anxiety disorders.

There are several treatments available for insomnia that can help improve mood and sleep quality. These treatments may include lifestyle changes, such as establishing a consistent sleep schedule and creating a relaxing bedtime routine, as well as medications.

It is important to address insomnia and mood changes as soon as possible to prevent them from worsening and affecting overall health and well-being.

Physical symptoms: Insomnia can also cause physical symptoms such as headaches, muscle tension, and gastrointestinal issues.

Dry mouth and throat: Waking up frequently or sleeping with your mouth open can lead to dryness in the mouth and throat.

Decreased appetite: Insomnia can cause changes in appetite and weight.

Increased risk of accidents: Insomnia can lead to impaired judgment and coordination, increasing the risk of accidents.

Increased risk of certain health conditions:
Chronic insomnia has been linked to an increased risk of certain health conditions, such as high blood pressure, heart disease, and diabetes.

CHAPTER 3

DIAGNOSIS OF INSOMNIA

There are several different types of insomnia, including acute insomnia, which is temporary and often caused by stress or other temporary factors; chronic insomnia, which is ongoing and may be caused by underlying medical or psychiatric conditions; and comorbid insomnia, which occurs in conjunction with other medical or psychiatric conditions.

To diagnose insomnia, a healthcare provider will typically conduct a thorough evaluation, including a medical history and physical examination, as well as a sleep history and a review of the patient's symptoms. The healthcare provider may also ask the patient to keep a sleep diary for several weeks, in which the patient records their sleep habits and any symptoms they experience.

In some cases, the healthcare provider may recommend a sleep study, also known as a polysomnogram, to assess the patient's sleep patterns and determine the cause of the insomnia. During a sleep study, the patient sleeps in a sleep lab or at home while wearing sensors that measure various aspects of their sleep, including brain activity, eye movements, muscle activity, and heart rate. The results of the sleep study can help the healthcare provider identify any underlying sleep disorders, such as sleep apnea, that may be contributing to the insomnia.

Other diagnostic tests may also be used to rule out or confirm other medical or psychiatric conditions that may be causing the insomnia. These tests may include blood tests, imaging studies, or psychological assessments.

Once the cause of the insomnia has been determined, the healthcare provider will recommend a treatment plan based on the specific needs of the patient. Treatment options for insomnia may include lifestyle changes, such as improving sleep habits and reducing stress; medication; or therapy, such as cognitive behavioral therapy for insomnia (CBT-I).

Lifestyle changes that may be recommended for people with insomnia include establishing a consistent sleep schedule, creating a relaxing bedtime routine, and avoiding stimulating activities before bedtime. It may also be helpful to avoid caffeine, alcohol, and large meals close to bedtime, and to get regular exercise during the day.

Medications that may be used to treat insomnia include sedatives, such as benzodiazepines and nonbenzodiazepine hypnotics, as well as melatonin agonists and antihistamines. These medications can be effective in helping people fall asleep, but they may have side effects, such as dizziness, dry mouth, and next-day grogginess, and they can be habit-forming.

Cognitive behavioral therapy for insomnia (CBT-I) is a form of therapy that focuses on helping people change negative thought patterns and behaviors that may be contributing to their insomnia. CBT-I typically involves a series of sessions with a therapist, in which the patient learns techniques for improving sleep habits and managing stress, and works to identify and modify any negative thoughts or behaviors that may be impacting their sleep.

Overall, the diagnosis and treatment of insomnia requires a comprehensive approach that considers the individual needs and circumstances of the patient. By working with a healthcare provider and taking an active role in their treatment, people with insomnia can often find relief from their symptoms and improve their overall quality of life.

CHAPTER 4

TREATMENT OF INSOMNIA

Treatment for insomnia often begins with lifestyle changes, as these can often be effective in improving sleep. Some of the lifestyle changes that may be recommended include:

- Establishing a regular sleep schedule: Going to bed and waking up at the same time every day can help regulate the body's sleep-wake cycle and improve sleep quality.

- Creating a relaxing bedtime routine: Doing activities like reading, taking a warm bath, or listening to calming music can help relax the body and mind and prepare them for sleep.

- Avoiding stimulants: Caffeine, nicotine, and electronics with screens (such as TVs, laptops, and smartphones) can stimulate

the brain and make it harder to fall asleep.
It is best to avoid these things for several
hours before bedtime.

- Making changes to the sleep environment:
  A comfortable mattress and pillows, a
  cool and dark bedroom, and white noise
  can all help create a more conducive sleep
  environment.

- Avoid stimulating activities before bed:
  Avoid screens (such as TVs, computers,
  and smartphones) for at least an hour
  before bed, as the blue light they emit can
  disrupt your sleep.

- Exercise during the day: Regular physical
  activity can help improve your sleep, but
  try to avoid vigorous exercise close to
  bedtime.

- Try relaxation techniques: There are a
  number of techniques that can help you

relax, such as deep breathing, meditation, or progressive muscle relaxation.

- Consider using sleep aids: If you've tried these strategies and are still struggling with insomnia, you may want to consider using over-the-counter or prescription sleep aids. However, it's important to use these products with caution, as they can have side effects and may not be suitable for long-term use.

There are also several types of medications that can help with insomnia. These include sedative-hypnotics, which are designed to help people fall asleep, and non-benzodiazepine hypnotics, which are less habit-forming than traditional sedative-hypnotics. Antidepressants and antihistamines may also be used to treat insomnia, although they are generally not as effective as sedative-hypnotics.

- Sedative-hypnotics are medications that are specifically designed to help people fall asleep. These include medications like benzodiazepines, which work by enhancing the effects of a neurotransmitter called GABA in the brain, and non-benzodiazepine hypnotics, which work in a similar way but are less likely to be habit-forming.

- Antidepressants and antihistamines may also be used to treat insomnia, although they are generally not as effective as sedative-hypnotics. Antidepressants work by altering the levels of certain chemicals in the brain, while antihistamines work by blocking the effects of histamine, a chemical that is involved in the sleep-wake cycle.

It is important to note that all medications have the potential for side effects and should only be taken under the supervision of a healthcare professional. It is also important to follow the recommended dosage and to not take any medication for an extended period of time without consulting a healthcare professional. Insomnia can often be managed through lifestyle changes, such as maintaining a consistent sleep schedule, creating a relaxing bedtime routine, and avoiding caffeine and screens before bedtime.

In addition to medication, there are several other treatment options for insomnia. Cognitive-behavioral therapy for insomnia (CBT-I) is a form of therapy that helps people change their thoughts and behaviors around sleep. It can be effective in improving sleep habits and reducing the severity of insomnia.

Other treatment options for insomnia include relaxation techniques, such as meditation and deep breathing, and exercise, which can help reduce stress and improve sleep quality. Some people find relief from insomnia by using natural remedies, such as herbal teas or supplements, although the effectiveness of these remedies has not been extensively studied.

It is important to note that insomnia is often a symptom of an underlying problem, and treating the underlying cause can help improve sleep. For example, if insomnia is caused by a medical condition, such as asthma or chronic pain, treating the condition may improve sleep. Similarly, if insomnia is caused by a medication, switching to a different medication or adjusting the dosage may help.

If lifestyle changes and medication do not improve insomnia, it is important to speak with a healthcare provider. In some cases, referral to a sleep specialist may be necessary. A sleep specialist can help identify the cause of the insomnia and develop a treatment plan tailored to the individual's needs.

In conclusion, insomnia is a common sleep disorder that can have a significant impact on daily functioning. Treatment for insomnia may involve lifestyle changes, medication, therapy, relaxation techniques, and addressing any underlying causes. It is important to speak with a healthcare provider if insomnia persists despite attempts to address it, as a sleep specialist may be able to help identify the cause and develop a treatment plan.

CHAPTER 5

COPING WITH INSOMNIA

Learning relaxation techniques

There are many relaxation techniques that can help with insomnia. Here are a few options:

Progressive muscle relaxation: This technique involves tensing and relaxing different muscle groups in the body, starting with the feet and working up to the head. The idea is to help the body relax and let go of tension.

Deep breathing: Taking slow, deep breaths can help calm the mind and body. One technique is to breathe in through the nose for a count of four, hold the breath for a count of four, and then exhale through the mouth for a count of four.

Guided imagery: This technique involves using the imagination to visualize a peaceful, calming scene or experience. This can help relax the mind and body and promote sleep.

Meditation: Meditation involves focusing the mind on a particular object, thought, or activity to train attention and awareness. It can help reduce stress and improve sleep.

Yoga or gentle stretching: Engaging in gentle physical activity, such as yoga or stretching, can help relax the body and mind and improve sleep.

It's important to find the relaxation technique that works best for you and to practice it regularly, especially before bedtime. It may also be helpful to create a bedtime routine that includes relaxation techniques as part of the routine.

Setting realistic sleep goals
Setting realistic sleep goals can be an important part of managing insomnia. Here are a few tips for setting and achieving sleep goals:

Start small: Rather than trying to overhaul your entire sleep routine all at once, start by making small changes. For example, you might aim to go to bed 15 minutes earlier each night or to limit caffeine consumption after a certain time.

Be consistent: Consistency is key when it comes to sleep. Try to go to bed and wake up at the same time every day, even on weekends. This can help regulate your body's natural sleep-wake cycle.

Make sleep a priority: Try to prioritize sleep in your daily routine. Create a bedtime routine that includes relaxation techniques and other activities that help you wind down before sleep.

Don't stress over sleep: It's important to remember that everyone's sleep needs are different, and it's normal to have occasional insomnia. Try not to stress or worry too much about not getting enough sleep, as this can actually make insomnia worse.

Seek professional help: If you're having trouble achieving your sleep goals or if your insomnia persists despite trying self-help measures, consider seeking professional help. A doctor or sleep specialist can help you identify any underlying causes of your insomnia and develop a treatment plan.

Seeking support from friends and family

Seeking support from friends and family can be an important part of managing insomnia. Here are a few ways that friends and family can support you:

Encourage healthy sleep habits: Encourage your loved ones to help you establish a consistent sleep routine and create a comfortable sleep environment.

Offer emotional support: Insomnia can be emotionally draining, and it's important to have a supportive network of friends and family to lean on. Let your loved ones know how you're feeling and ask for their emotional support.

Help with tasks: Insomnia can make it difficult to complete everyday tasks, and it can be helpful to have loved ones pitch in. Consider asking for help with household chores or errands to free up time for rest and relaxation.

Encourage you to seek professional help: If your insomnia persists despite trying self-help measures, it may be helpful to seek professional help. Encourage your loved ones to support you in seeking treatment from a doctor or sleep specialist.

It's important to remember that everyone's sleep needs are different, and it's normal to have occasional insomnia. Don't be afraid to reach out to friends and family for support when you need it.

Seeking professional help (such as seeing a therapist or doctor)

If you're having trouble managing your insomnia despite trying self-help measures, it may be helpful to seek professional help. Here are a few options for seeking professional help for insomnia:

Seeing a doctor: A primary care doctor or a sleep specialist can help identify any underlying medical conditions that may be contributing to your insomnia and recommend treatment options.

Seeing a therapist: A therapist or counselor can help you identify and address any psychological or emotional issues that may be contributing to your insomnia. They may recommend cognitive-behavioral therapy (CBT) for insomnia, which is a type of therapy that helps people change negative thoughts and behaviors that can interfere with sleep.

Taking medication: In some cases, a doctor may recommend medication to help improve sleep. There are several types of medications that can be used to treat insomnia, including sedative-hypnotics, melatonin agonists, and tricyclic antidepressants. It's important to discuss the potential risks and benefits of medication with a doctor before starting any new medication.

It's important to remember that everyone's sleep needs are different, and what works for one person may not work for another. If you're considering seeking professional help for your insomnia, it's a good idea to talk to a doctor or therapist to discuss your options and find a treatment plan that's right for you.

CONCLUSION AND NEXT STEPS
In the conclusion of this guide on insomnia, it's important to do as saids in this book and follow this keys

Make positive changes: I encourage you to take the steps you've learned about, such as establishing a consistent bedtime routine, creating a comfortable sleep environment, and seeking professional help if needed.

Follow up with a healthcare provider: I encourage you to follow up with a healthcare provider if your insomnia persists or if you have concerns about your sleep.

Stay positive: I encourage you to stay positive and remember that everyone's sleep needs are different, and it's normal to have occasional insomnia. You need to find the strategies that work for you and be patient as you work to improve your sleep.

In conclusion, insomnia is a common sleep disorder that can have negative impacts on physical and mental health. There are many strategies and treatment options available for managing insomnia, and it's important to find what works best for an individual's needs. With the right approach, it is possible to improve sleep and lead a healthier, more fulfilling life.

RECAP OF KEYPOINTS
Here is a recap of the key points about insomnia:

- Insomnia is a sleep disorder characterized by difficulty falling asleep, staying asleep, or both.
- Insomnia can have negative impacts on physical and mental health, including increased risk of accidents, decreased productivity, and negative effects on mood and mental health.
- There are many factors that can contribute to insomnia, including stress, anxiety, certain medications, and certain medical conditions.
- There are several treatment options for insomnia, including lifestyle changes, behavioral therapies, and medications.
- Improving sleep hygiene and practicing relaxation techniques can be helpful in managing insomnia.
- If self-help measures are not sufficient, seeking professional help from a doctor or therapist may be necessary.
- Everyone's sleep needs are different, and it's important to find what works best for an individual's needs.

Printed in Great Britain
by Amazon

18232873R00047